Contribution of ultrasound to inflammatory
abdominal disease

Radiological study

I0483024

Constantin Panow

Printed by CreateSpace

*"There are in fact two things, science and opinion,
the former begets knowledge, the latter ignorance".
Hippocrates (460-370BC)*

## Contents

*Key words*

Abdominal ultrasound; diagnosis of abdominal infections; radiological diagnosis; non-invasive diagnosis for ulcer disease; inflammation of bowel.

Ultrasound has been devoted to medical tasks since end of World War 2. (1950, Glasgow)

In its origins it has been developed by allied scientists in order to track German submarines;

Once a nightmare for sea transportation at the beginning of World War 2.

Soon after beginning of use of powerful sonars in American fleet, German submariners suffered a true disaster.

This profile of German navy was literally destroyed, suffering a loss of almost 95% in only a few months.

After end of War, scientific acquisitions were oriented to peaceful applications, in Medicine for instance.

At first abdominal ultrasound was able to diagnose only gallbladder stones.

With better image processing, resolution and hard disc space and faster analysis, other medical topics could be tracked with success.

It is at the turn of the Century, somewhere 1998 or 1999;

That ultrasound machines, called also echographs, benefited completely from the computer revolution;

And acquired performances, which made them able to sustain true comparison with other radiological modalities, be it MRI or scannography.

At that time, the two biggest Mega-Konzerne (Huge firms), which are still main actors in Radiology;

Siemens acquiring Acuson, and Philips, buying ATL;

Were main competitors on the Market;

Proposing for the first time machines able to multiply several times previously attained capabilities in all tasks.

This reality is by no way old history;

As thus attained image quality would need not years, but tens of years;

To be described in medical literature, with its following applications;

And consequences for patients, doctors and medical authority.

Promoting not only better analysis and diagnosis of medical entities;

But adding to existing knowledge in all directions, even therapy.

Missing literature is still one main problem, as physicians from other specialties are unable to follow development of technology, and frequently do not believe diagnoses obtained by ultrasound.

There are several explanations to this issue:

The first is reimbursement policy of modern insurance companies, which discard by low price ultrasound as effective means to diagnosis.

This is very unfortunate, as echographs are not only inexpensive as technology;

They are also very effective way of work up in many situations, and sometimes - the only one.

Second problem is training in this modality:

If scanner and MRI are claimed to be *reproducible* techniques, while ultrasound - examiner dependent;

Modern evolution and practice show, that all techniques, even simplest X-Ray are *examiner dependent!*

What all modern imagery taught us, is that X-Ray depicts many more details, than what was previously believed or claimed to be standard;

And future belongs to inexpensive and efficient techniques, not to expensive ones.

Many authorities claim, that a resident in Radiology is trained with only one single year practice in MRI or scanner.

For ultrasound, this is by no way accurate, as it needs many years to become proficient at it.

Difficulty in this modality lies not only in interpretation of image, but also in its acquisition.

Third point: Available literature by no way describes correctly state of the art: - its position limping not years, but tens of years back in the past.

Fourth feature: Increasing prevalence of viral disease on the Planet;

Main reason for this observation being increasing ease of transportation, responsible for a huge mixing and brewing of viral layout on the Planet;

People being exposed to genuine infection, with which their immune system has never been in touch before.

This issue makes every specialist in training reluctant to spend time in learning a technology, which makes him ill all the time.

Because every other discipline limits contact with patients to a minimum:

A big desk in between;

Short physical examination.

But if you want to be proficient with ultrasound, you need to implement one extra parameter, which is time;

In direct contact with the patient, breathing same air as him/her.

Fifth problem resides in practice of medicine all over the world.

As training and investment on the part of physicians increases, with volume and complexity of teaching, and time devoted to study of the subject;

The public becomes reluctant at paying for health services;

Resulting in fewer candidates for this hard profession.

There is a chronic deficit in medical doctors all over the Planet.

This observation goes hand in hand with change in philosophy of training.

Once, physicians would start with an interview of every patient;

And would proceed further to physical examination after strict rules of their profession;

Laboratory and radiological exams coming only next in such programmed schedule.

Today we joke:

That if MRI (Magic Radiological Imagery) would not provide us with a diagnosis, we would proceed to questioning the patient.

Discipline is no more warranted in profession of *Asclepius*.

Anything is good to do or to ask.

Once doctors would learn signs and symptoms of disease.

Nowadays they believe blindly in virtues of laboratory;

The more complicated and costly the exam, the more they are lulled in ordering it.

I remember 35 years ago, as a young practitioner, I would write on every file my diagnosis, be it measles or rubella, without any blood exam;

Nowadays colleagues are completely unable to diagnose *measles* after its signs and symptoms;

They order an antibody search instead;

Costly, taking time, and even not always correct;

As there is a rate of false negatives which plagues every single exam;

Professors of medicine invent new diseases and entities, which exist only in their imagination:

As for example: - *fibromyalgia* and *dyspepsia*.

As to second, I refer you to the excellent work by Jerome K. Jerome: *Three men in a boat and other stories.*

> *It explains you precisely what we should think about the term dyspepsia in its most comedian analysis.*

*As to first entity, I could never witness a single case of it during my practice of more than 30 years. Instead I could coin a different diagnosis on each file reporting such disease.*

Of course, those excellent colleagues are unable to understand, that a physician can diagnose measles with just a few questions and a short exam.

As my practice is issued from medical philosophy established almost half a century ago;

They are unable to follow my reasoning and understand;

That I am able in the same way of thinking to coin a specific germ, responsible for illness after an ultrasound examination.

Nobody knows anymore who *Fiessinger, Leroy and Reiter* were.

People do not even believe, that there is a rationale behind this entity, described in the years of World War 1.

Because means of examination at that time were to their appreciation insufficient to pinpoint such a disease.

Public forgets how inventions of science happen:

Charles Darwin, for instance, describes for the first time frame of evolution of species as such. (1859)

For this task he is using a microscope (Appears in late 16<sup>th</sup> century, in Netherlands) and a magnifying glass (First mentioned 424 BC, in Aristophanes joke);

In fact, for accuracy sake, he is using much more second, than first.

Both invented centuries before.

As for Louis Pasteur, he proves 1864, by a simple procedure, proliferation of microbes;

Vents away all opposition to the *germ theory*;

And invents *pasteurization* for milk and other alimentary products, still in use today.

Again, he is using technical acquisitions present since centuries.

Italian glass making was able to produce devices used by Pasteur since 14<sup>th</sup> century (Murano).

Thus, in contradistinction to modern appreciation, scientific discoveries are not determined by technological means;

But rather by simple methodology and application of thinking in a logical way, in the frame of a decent discipline.

*Brain work, being limiting factor in progress of science, as to what History provides us with examples.*

What concerns my practice in diagnostic ultrasound, my philosophy derives from medical training as general practitioner:

I start with anamnesis, which proceeds in an uninterrupted pattern through every examination, pertinent questions being implemented in an informal way;

Ultrasound image is prolongation of my fingers and main instrument, but every information thus collected is verified with *physical status*;

As pathology can be described on every picture, but clinical signs are as important for diagnosis.

I use to joke with my patients, that in contradistinction to my colleagues from veterinary medicine, my patients talk.

And I use this feature.

*A nice image alone permits not more than 50-60% of diagnoses!*

This ratio jumping way above 90% with pertinent questioning and examination.

A beautiful image can be not pertinent to diagnosis at all;

While a poor quality image could be addressed and improved to valuable information with palpatory supplementation.

And I joke sometimes with my patients, who ask me how I can see something on such a device:

*It is the same way as society of women:*

*A beautiful one is not necessarily helpful;*

*While a less good looking one can be not only entertaining, but even educative!*

As to practical pattern of examination, already 30 years ago, specialists of sonography would establish the useful postulate, that you need to examine gallbladder in two different positions;

Either recumbent and upright, or some other mixture and modification of those two.

Standing position needs a complete change in examination technique;

And as such, I seldom resort to it, unless I have to do with inguinal or femoral herniation, which are not visible with Valsalva maneuvers.

Infrequently I apply this technique also in a case of gastro-duodenal ulceration, which is not visible in lying position on the couch.

Or in whatever condition, which can be diagnosed only by a complete change of examination pattern.

As a rule, I do every abdominal ultrasound in three different positions:

Flat:

But if I say:

"Turn on your back", people would turn on their tummy in 90% of cases.

In left recumbent situation, and right lateral position.

Precision being necessary for left or right orders;

Because, though all patients that I examine have attended obligatory school, they are frequently unable to show their right or left side;

So, I say: *Towards the wall!*

To which also some have another objection: *Which one?*

And if I say: *Turn on the other side!*

My patient would ask again: - *Which one?*

As to philosophical interpretation of this frame of logic in general population;

The only reference I could find is from Revelation, last book of the Bible;

Where the author claims, that Archangels (*Living Creatures*) have several sides;

And that they are able to move in several directions at the same time...

Let's start with examples:

*Gastro-duodenal ulceration*

Once believed to result from acidity produced in the stomach;

Propagated as utter truth not far away from today, only in the mid 1970ties.

Now we know it is due to bacterial infection.

In 95% of cases *Helicobacter pylori*.

Hosted by 97% of population on Earth.

In 1- 5% of cases due to some other germ of gastro-intestinal tract;

Most of the time *Campylobacter jejuni*, as this is, or has been most frequent pathogen in last 20years.

But, there are still some colleagues who haven't grasped that truth;

And would treat their patients not with antibiotics;

But with gastric anti-secretory medication;

And would even be astonished, that it doesn't work.

As to history, Helicobacter disease invented by Australian scientists in the 1980ties is by no way a quite genuine discovery.

As History goes;

America has been discovered several times.

In early 1970ties, there was a professor of Radiology at the University Hospital of Bern, Switzerland, who would describe *gastro-duodenal ulcers* with double contrast barium examination.

(Professor Adolf Zuppinger, Titularprofessor am Inselspital, Bern since 1947.)

In order to distinguish benign from malignant disease, he would order Tetracycline therapy for two weeks, and repeat barium exam.

If it still showed the ulcer, it was claimed to be malignant, otherwise- benign.

As this shows, knowledge about infectious etiology of gastric ulcer, was already old, when Australian scientists Barry Marschall and Robin Warren described this principle, together with *Helicobacter pylori* disease.(1982)

As to future development in the field, it is already at your door;

Peaking like a flower in my garden;

I observe, that acidity and Helicobacter pylori infection are not enough, as gastro-duodenal ulcer opens often with viral infection.

Remains to establish which kind;

Is it more frequently Norovirus or Rotavirus, for instance?

And in a few years, we would treat it not with antibiotics, but with antivirals.

Apart from these features, it is a chronic disease;

A visit to the gastroenterologists' office wouldn't always be able to establish it.

The ulcer can stay open for two weeks, then close, and not recur for years.

It is strongly determined by stress, be it professional or in the realm of family.

Not everybody can develop this disease, but genetic predisposition has not yet been described, apart from blood group; (to my knowledge)

Most people, suffering from it, are either group O or A.

Only very seldom I would have a patient with group AB, and even rarer B.

Also acidity, as claimed previously, is not totally independent from pathophysiology of this disease.

Modern treatment proposes gastric anti-secretory drugs in association with antibiotics.

Modern ultrasound machines provide reliable image of this disease in a very high percentage of cases.

It is sufficient to know where to look, and how to do it.

Ulcers are most of the time tiny, measuring between 1 and 3 mm; (0,04 to 0,12 inches)

Most frequently on wall of duodenal bulbus (75% about), and less frequently in gastric antrum (Approximately 25% in my series).

They are most easily visible in left recumbent position, and you can see them already with a curved probe (5-2 MHz).

As far, as corpulence of my patient permits, I try to obtain a high resolution image with a flat probe (12-5 MHz).

Palpatory examination at the same time with the probe is mandatory, as it allows to determinate whether thus obtained image is linked to patients' pain;

And second, but not last, whether this person consults precisely for this ailment.

Application of probe tightly to the spot, where you see suggestive image permits to answer those two questions.

It is essential for clarity's sake to separate those two topics, as most patients are unable to answer both questions with first essay.

Trying several times, and establishing a good relationship with your patient helps tremendously your diagnostic process.

Jokes have also an important part in this procedure, as relaxation of mind and body are essential part of discussion.

Any stress implemented by you, your white blouse, or the patient, himself, or herself, can impede with this process, and false your diagnosis.

This is especially the case with children, who are anxious, because of previous contact with doctors;

I tell them:

*I am not a doctor!*

*I neither cut, not prick;*

*I am just a photographer;*

*We are going to make a picture of your tummy;*

*Do you like pictures?*

*Can you smile for it?*

Most laugh;

If they are big enough.

If the stomach is empty, antral ulcers can be diagnosed almost in all parts of this structure;

As to bulbar ulcers, most difficult location is posterior;

Anamnesis is essential in this case, as antral location never causes back pain, which is the rule for bulbar site of disease.

Thoroughness of examination is, needless to say, main objective;

Most ulcers are located on upper wall of antrum or bulbus, according to *micro-aerophilic properties* of this germ. (Necessitating air to multiply)

Frequent variations of this main position are anterior wall, then posterior.

As to relative percentages:

*Bulbar ulcer:*

50% superior wall;

30% anterior;

20% posterior;

Inferior location is exceptional.

*Antral ulcers* have similar statistical distribution.

Most ulcers on anterior or posterior wall locate in *upper part* of it.

Ultrasound permits you also to determine whether this lesion is limited to stomach or duodenal wall, its extension and depth;

And whether it *is transfixiating*;

In which case you can have also a tiny film of *ascites* along gallbladder, pancreas and stomach and duodenum.

Excluding gallbladder disease;

And even more difficult, pancreas involvement are essential *aims of this task*.

As to determining whether Helicobacter pylori is responsible for disease;

As it is proposed by so- called specialists;

It is a problem of simple statistical calculation, which is taught to most doctors practicing internal medicine.

I can only wonder that this topic never reached cells of grey matter to which it was addressed...

As with any exam, there is a percentage of false negatives;

For most types of examination searching for Helicobacter, sensitivity is between 65 and 85%.

*A priori* probability to deal with this infection, as already mentioned, is 97%.

A positive test would lift this ratio above 99%;

While a negative test would lower it somewhere in 90% probability.

Many practitioners would treat only patients with a positive test, neglecting this kind of simple mathematics. (Bayes' theorem)

It is worthwhile mentioning it, as medical doctors are the first to complain about shortening of coverage.

*Campylobacter*

Ultrasound can also tackle this specific topic;

As next most frequently encountered germ is *Campylobacter jejuni.*

*Campylobacter jejuni infection of bowel.*

A few years ago this was the most frequent bacterial infection caused by ingestion of raw or poorly cooked meat.

In Swiss butcher shops 70% of poultry, pork and sheep meat, and 50% of veal, beef and lamb are infected with germs.

Intestinal infection produces a very specific image on ultrasound examination:

Bowel thickening;

As with any bacterial agent, is superior to what is seen with most viral agents;

And is at least 3mm in thickness (0,12 inches);

Be it *distal small bowel*, most typical location;

Or thick bowel, most frequent location being *sigmoid colon*.

*Gastritis* caused by this agent is less common, but opening of ulcer in predisposed population has been described many years ago.

Typical feature is reaction *of lymph nodes*:

They are multiple;

Located either *in right lower quadrant*;

Or less commonly in *left lower mesenterium*;

Usually *multiple*;

Well seen with a flat probe;

Depicting 5 to 10 such nodes per field (4,4 cm probe; 1,73 inches length);

Main characteristic of this infection is, that they are all almost *same size*;

6 to 7 mm maximal length. (0,24 to 0,28 inches)

In recent years ingestion of raw meat, as for instance a steak, cooked rare, causes another frequent infection, which was exceptional in such a case 10 years ago:

*Listeria monocytogenes*.

Ten years ago I would observe this infectious agent only in the case of ingestion of salami, or other uncooked appetizers, and rarely with cheese (Camembert, for instance- soft heart variant).

Its features on ultrasound:

Bowel thickening even more prominent, than with Campylobacter species (>3mm-0.12 inches).

Most frequent location being caecum and ileum.

Characteristic lymph node reaction is also present:

3 to 8 mesenteric lymph nodes per field. (4,4 cm probe; 1,73 inches length)

*Highly variable size* of lymph nodes:

Between 4 and 18 mm in maximal diameter (0.16 to 0.71 inches).

Most frequent location being *right lower quadrant*.

As to utility of this diagnosis:

This being pretty obvious;

The only possible means to determine type of infectious agent, is bacterial culture of stool.

Positive diagnosis with this examination is about 80% on the first day of disease;

Sinking continually with duration of infection, being in vicinity of 40% the second day, and only 20% the third day;

A positive diagnosis after 4th day with this procedure is exceptional.

As most patients consult from 3rd day onwards, advantage of alternative procedure for diagnosis becomes evident;

In future, laboratories could provide us with a PCR test, which would be a big progress;

Unfortunately we do not dispose yet with this possibility.

Questioning the patient about previous meal;

Usually just 2 – 3 hours before outbreak of pain, and/or diarrhea;

Should be placed on same level of importance as ultrasound image;

And *anamnesis* is probably as reliable for diagnosis as ultrasound itself!

*Escherichia coli*

Less frequently acquired pathogens following consumption of raw meat are Escherichia coli.

In fact its frequency is growing;

Making up only 20-30% 10 years ago;

It reaches now almost 40- 50% of cases.

Involvement of different parts of bowel is highly variable;

Being able to concern whole gastro-intestinal tract from stomach to anus.

Thickening of bowel wall is at least 3 mm; (0,12 inches)

Lymph node reaction *is inconspicuous*.

*Vibrio species*

Less common pathogens:

*Vibrio para-haemolyticus* and haemolyticus:

Due to ingestion of *raw sea food*;

Bowel wall thickening is variable, but not prominent;

In vicinity of 3 mm most of the time; (<0,12 inches)

Splenomegaly (Light; > 350ml volume) is present in 50% of cases;

Lymph node reaction is prominent;

1 – 3 lymph nodes per field. (4,4 cm probe; 1,73 inches length)

*Slightly variable size*;

Maximal diameter oscillating between 6 and 12 mm. (0.24 to 0.47 inches)

*Salmonella species*

Exceptional in Western Europe:

Most cases in our facility being acquired in the Middle East.

Infection can be protracted;

Frequently of low aggressiveness;

Bowel thickening is less conspicuous; (<<3mm)

Lymph nodes are well visible;

2- 6 per field; (4,4 cm probe; 1,73 inches length)

Size is *stable, and small;*

4 to 5 mm maximal diameter. (0.16 to 0.2 inches)

The agent of cat scratch fever, *Bartonella henselae*:

Very atypical bowel disease;

Lymph node reaction being most prominent:

Few lymph nodes are present in mesentery;

Usually only 1 to 5 in total number;

*Size is prominent, almost huge*;

In vicinity of 2 to 3.5 cm (0.78 to 1.37 inches).

Necrosis is frequently visible.

Nodes are hyper-vascular on *doppler*.

Thickening of bowel wall is variable, depending on duration of disease, present at first, then less and less conspicuous.

Pseudo-membranous colitis:

Due to *Clostridium difficile* infection;

After prescription of antibiotics;

Could be much more frequent, than supposed;

Usually well visible in sigmoid colon;

As important thickening of bowel wall (>5mm-0.2 inches)

Loosening of wall texture is prominent feature (Hence pseudo-membranes observed at endoscopy).

Mesenteric lymph node reaction is not conspicuous.

Several similar agents can be involved;

*Mycobacterium tuberculosis:*

Once prevalent on the Old Continent:

Then spread by colonization all over the World:

Eradicated in industrialized countries with beginning of 20$^{th}$ century;

At first with sun-baths and better living conditions:

Warmed homes; three meals per day;

Then with *anti-microbials*;

Now this germ is becoming resistant to antibiotics, because of irrational use of those;

It involves only seldom the gastro-intestinal tract;

Unless it is *Mycobacterium bovis:*

The infection of which is promoted by drinking un-pasteurized milk.

Sometimes the result of alimentary faddism;

It produces ascites, as in lungs, where pleura is frequently involved;

In abdomen, peritoneal layers participate commonly in disease;

Mesenteric lymph node reaction is typical;

Lymph nodes are numerous;

And of intermediate size;

Variability of maximal diameter is between 4 and 8 mm(0.16 to 0.31 inches)

Diagnosis is difficult, because of rarity of disease;

*Nobody thinks about this possibility!*

Certification of germ must be aimed with laparoscopy and analysis of nodes or peritoneal plaques.

Participation of liver and spleen is late occurrence;

Thickening of bowel wall is not observed, as infection is most of the time protracted, and examined with radiological means only in its late stadium.

*Atypical mycobacteria* are commonly encountered in AIDS infection:

*Mycobacteria avium intra-cellulare complex* or MAC:

Can also involve on rare occasions intestines:

Diagnosis is easy in this context;

As lymph nodes are big;

In vicinity of 2 to 3 cm (0.79 to 1.2 inches);

And with hypo-dense center on scanner.

*Whipple disease:*

Due to *Tropheryma whippeli:*

Rare bacterial infection;

Can involve whole small bowel, predominantly;

Stomach and thick bowel being less concerned;

Ileum is common site;

Lymph node reaction is prominent;

1 – 3 lymph nodes per field of view (4,4 cm probe; 1,73 inches length)

Size moderately variable;

4- 8 mm maximal diameter most of the time;

Thickening of small bowel can be in excess of 3 mm.

A differential diagnosis of mesenteric lymphadenopathy in childhood might be gluten intolerance.

Lymph nodes in this ailment tend to be less numerous, than in infectious disease, and there is no excess of fluid content in small bowel, as it uses to be in case of infection.

Variability of lymph nodes is moderate, usually 5-12 mm (0.19-0.47 inches) in maximal diameter.

With linear high resolution probe you see usually not more than 1-3 such structures per view.

They are located in right iliac fossa, but can distribute evenly in all small bowel mesentery.

*Hiatal herniation*

And its inflammation:

Most common cause of abdominal aches;

At first in epigastric location, at night;

In recumbent position;

Irradiating in right hypochondrium being common;

In left hypochondrium, - also possible;

Extending after a few days over whole abdomen;

Due most of the time to viral disease;

Making up almost 80% of consultations for abdominal ultrasound;

Because 50% of population is at risk;

Due to deficient anti-reflux mechanism;

Manifesting itself after weight gain;

Well visible on ultrasound;

The best picture being obtained in left lateral decubitus position;

And in *inspiration*;

Typical image is a double gastro-esophageal junction;

Once the real one;

And a second time a false one, situated distally to the first;

Giving to this part of tract the typical appearance *of irregular conformation*;

Frequently reflux itself is visible during examination;

Thickening of bowel wall at this place is frequently above 5mm; (0.2 inches)

Though etiology is viral;

(+ Acid);

Involving not only distal esophagus, as you would think after reading books on the subject;

But even proximal stomach wall;

Frequently attaining 8 mm, (0.31 inches);

Without having Boerhaave's disease; or Mallory-Weiss, nor Barrett's esophagus or whatsoever;

Confirmed by gentle pressure on this junction with the probe, in inspiration;

And asking the patient, first to confirm that it is painful;

And second to tell you, whether he/she consults precisely for this ache and ailment.

*Gastritis*

Can be viral or bacterial;

Or chronic;

That is autoimmune;

Thickening of 3 or more mm of stomach wall (0.12 inches);

Is to be considered bacterial;

Unless, there is also associated slight splenomegaly (350 to 550 ml),

In which case it is frequently due to infectious mononucleosis;

Ebstein-Barr disease;

In this entity even colon can be site of prominent infection;

And having thickened wall, accordingly;

But never above 3-3.5 mm (0.12 inches), like stomach.

The only viral disease producing bowel wall thickening in vicinity of 3 mm (0.12 inches);

And thus making it difficult to differentiate from bacterial infection.

Most enteric viral infections, (If not all) producing only thickening of mucosa;

Transverse thickness of bowel wall being less than 2 mm (0.078 inches).

*Diverticulitis*

Frequently reason for consultations;

Most prominent in left lower quadrant;

Involving more sigmoid colon, than any other segment;

Familial predisposition;

Usually chronic constipation is present since years;

Sometimes declares itself already in patients' 20ties;

Obese subjects are more frequently concerned;

Well visible with ultrasound in most patients;

Even when obese;

Confusion can occur if illness is chronic at time of consultation;

And has elicited bowel wall thickening, which can be prominent;

Difficult to distinguish from malignant disease;

Distinction is possible if involved segment is long;

More than 8 cm (3.1 inches);

And thickening of bowel wall less than 5 mm (0.2 inches);

In all other cases endoscopy is mandatory;

*Diverticula* are most of the time between 3 and 10 mm in diameter (0.12 -0.39 inches).

Recurring diverticulitis can be due to distal obstruction (Rectum or recto-sigmoid junction);

To be checked for, accordingly during examination;

Most adeno-carcinomas of colon being visible on ultrasound.

In contradistinction to what can be read on internet;

And has been taught in medical schools 40 years ago;

*It is **not due** to inflammation of appendix vermiformis!*

Which one can originate following any infectious agent whatsoever;

*But to **obstruction** of this blind ending portion of bowel!*

By thickened feces;

Sometimes by worms;

Its transverse diameter in this situation exceeds 1.5 cm (0.59 inches);

Most of the time in vicinity of 1.7 cm (0.67 inches) in adult population;

When obstruction is acute;

1.4 cm (0.55 inches) or less in diameter can mean, either that you are on the site of progression of disease;

Or more frequently on the down-slope of spontaneous resolution;

That is, the plug has loosened;

Which happens in 90% of cases;

Only 10% of those perforate;

And cause peritonitis;

Which is invariably the situation when there is free ascites;

*Another reason for misunderstanding of this topic!*

Perforation happens most of the time with oozing of pus from the appendix;

When it is frank, with a hole, it frequently kills the patient on the spot;

Because of septic shock!

Thickening of appendix wall is sign for duration of disease;

Acute appendicitis evolves in a time frame of 24 hours or 2- 3 days;

Without appropriate treatment, it usually kills within a week, since first signs;

When perforation in peritoneal cavity occurs;

This disease is still lethal in our highly medicated society!

And further main provider of patients with recurrent intestinal occlusions;

Several excellent publications have shown in recent literature that ultrasound is suited as best modality for such diagnosis:

I would depict only a few of these, in order to fill a breach in pertinent information, already available;

Or *Enterobius vermicularis*:

Most frequent Nematode worm;

Rather than a parasite, it has symbiotic behavior with humans;

Essential for equilibrium of our immune system;

Its permanent eradication can cause autoimmune disease;

Present in every single human on the Planet!

Genetic renewal of population in bowels is substantiated by eating fresh salad;

As it is ubiquitous in earth all over the World;

Measures 0.7 to 0.9 mm in transverse diameter (0.027 to 0.035 inches);

Males measure 8 to 15 mm in length (0.31- 0.59 inches);

While females can measure up to 5 cm in length (2 inches);

Easy to diagnose with modern ultrasound machines accordingly.

Those worms cause seldom disease:

Most of the time in spring, when irradiation from the sun tells them, that it is high season;

They proliferate;

Can erode slightly small bowel wall;

And less frequently colon mucosa;

Cause slight pain in right iliac fossa;

Distal ileum is involved;

Another typical pathological case, is that worm females, which are long enough, can travel in feminine genitals;

And cause urethritis;

Typically manifests with dysuria, without pyuria, nor blood in urine;

Frequently recurrent;

Unless treated;

Can be diagnosed (Appropriate length of females) in sigmoid colon;

Transverse diameter of those attains 1 mm (0.04 inches)

One single anti-parasitic drug is sufficient to limit their population;

Long females need 2- 3 years to grow to their adult size.

Or *Strongyloides stercoralis:*

Another Nematode worm:

Having a true parasitic behavior to humans;

Its lung cycle makes it dangerous!

*Producing septic clinical image, even shock, without bacterial growth on blood cultures*;

Occasionally can be diagnosed on chest X-Ray, if typical pattern of *Loeffler's syndrome* is recognizable;

Also easy to diagnose on abdominal ultrasound;

Much smaller pathogen than *Enterobius*;

Measures 0.3-0.4 mm in transverse diameter (0.01 to 0.016 inches);

Length: between 5 and 8 mm usually (0.2 to 0.3 inches);

Most frequently can be shown in distal ileum;

Abdominal ultrasound is essential for diagnosis, as stool examination is typically unrevealing of present infection.

PCR could provide easier diagnosis in future.

## Summary Chart

| Inflammation type | Mesenteric lymph node (LN) reaction | Number of LN | LN size | Location |
|---|---|---|---|---|
| Campylobacter | Prominent | numerous | 7mm, stable | Ileum>colon |
| Listeria monocytogenes | Prominent | numerous | 4-15mm, variable | ileum>colon |
| Yersiniosis | Prominent | numerous | 6-8mm, -stable | ileum mainly |
| Salmonella | Less conspicuous | less prominent | 4-5mm, stable | ileum mainly |
| Whipple's dis. | can be prominent | variable | 5-8mm, +variable | small intestine |
| Vibrio para-haemol. | lesser extent | less numerous | 5-10mm, +variable | small intestine |
| Escherichia coli | inconspicuous | / | / | colon>ileum |
| Bartonella henselae | huge, prominent in Doppler vasc. | <2 or 3 | 2 to 3.5cm | small intestine |
| Clostridium difficile | inconspicuous | / | / | colon |
| Tuberculosis | prominent | numerous | 5-8mm, stable | ileum>colon |
| MAC | prominent | variable | 2-3cm, variable | diffuse |
| AINS/Aspirine intolerance | inconspicuous | / | / | colon, sigmoid |
| Arterial insufficiency | inconspicuous | / | / | sigmoid,desc. |
| Enterobius v. | inconspicuous | / | / | sigmoid,desc. |
| Diverticulitis | inconspicuous | / | / | sigmoid>rest of colon |
| Adenocarcinoma of colon | variable >3mm depends on grade | variable | variable, mets | rectum>sigmoid |
| Viral disease | inconspicuous | / | / | variable |
| Ebstein-Barr dis. | can be present | rare | small, 3mm | throughout |
| Gluten intolerance | can be present | can be numerous | 5-9mm, variable | ileum mainly |

| Inflammation type | Intestinal wall thickness |
|---|---|
| Campylobacter | >3.5mm |
| Listeria monocytogenes | >4mm |
| Yersiniosis | >3mm |
| Salmonella | <3.5mm |
| Whipple's dis. | <3.5mm |
| Vibrio para-haemol. | <3mm |
| Escherichia coli | >3mm |
| Bartonella henselae | >4mm |
| Clostridium difficile | 7mm |
| Tuberculosis | <3mm |
| MAC | >4mm |
| AINS/Aspirine intolerance | >2.5mm, mucosa |
| Arterial insufficiency | >2.5mm, mucosa |
| Enterobius v. | <2.5mm, mucosa |
| Diverticulitis | variable >3mm |
| Adenocarcinoma of colon | >1.5cm usually |
| Viral disease | <2mm, mucosa |
| Ebstein-Barr dis. | >2.5-3mm |
| Gluten intolerance | >2.5mm |

(USA measurement system)

| Inflammation type | LN size | Intestinal wall |
|---|---|---|
| Campylobacter | 0.28", stable | >0.14" |
| Listeria monocytogenes | 0.16-0.6", variable | >0.16" |
| Yersiniosis | 0.24-0.31", - stable | >0.12" |
| Salmonella | 0.16-0.2", stable | <0.14" |
| Whipple's dis. | 0.2-0.31", +variable | <0.14" |
| Vibrio para-haemol. | 0.2-0.4", +variable | <0.12" |
| Escherichia coli | / | >0.12" |
| Bartonella henselae | 0.79-1.6" | >0.16" |
| Clostridium difficile | / | 0.28" |
| Tuberculosis | 0.2-0.31 i, stable | <0.12" |
| MAC | 0.8-1.2 i, variable | >0.16" |
| AINS/Aspirine intolerance | / | >0.1", mucosa |

| | | |
|---|---|---|
| Arterial insufficiency | / | >0.1", mucosa |
| Enterobius v. | / | <0.1", mucosa |
| Diverticulitis | / | variable >0.12" |
| Adenocarcinoma of colon | variable, mets | >0.59" usually |
| Viral disease | / | <0.08", mucosa |
| Ebstein-Barr dis. | small, 0.12" | >0.1-0.12" |
| Gluten intolerance | 0.2-0.35", variable | >0.12" |

One of my previous chiefs in Radiology Department would joke in his retirement speech;

That:

*A dwarf on the shoulders of a giant sees further than the giant himself! ;*

(As his predecessor was a very famous Swiss radiologist);

And he would continue:

*But how about a giant on a giants' shoulders?*

I hope you enjoyed this short text.

If you find it helpful, please leave an evaluation in a few months or years.

If you do this more people would be able to apply my methods.

You can reach me at
*http://www.thenopillshealthprospect.com*

Or at:
*http://www.amazon.com/author/constantinpanow*

If you have any questions or comments, do not hesitate, write in my blog!

www.ingramcontent.com/pod-product-compliance
Lightning Source LLC
Chambersburg PA
CBHW071758170526
45167CB00003B/1085